Red Light Therapy for Youthful Complexion

DIY steps in unlocking the new
anti-aging secret for younger, beautiful
and radiant skin

By

James E. Philip's

TABLE OF CONTENT

Introduction to Red Light Therapy**: An overview of red light therapy, its history, and its scientific principles.

The history of red light therapy, also known as photobiomodulation therapy, is a captivating journey that spans over a century. From its humble beginnings as an experimental concept to its widespread adoption in modern medicine and wellness, the evolution of this therapeutic approach is nothing short of remarkable.

Early Pioneers: The Dawn of Light Therapy (1903-1960s)

The roots of red light therapy can be traced back to the early 20th century when visionary scientists began to explore the therapeutic potential of light. Notably, Niels Ryberg Finsen, a Danish physician, laid the foundation for the field. In 1903, Finsen was awarded the Nobel Prize in Physiology or Medicine for his pioneering work on the treatment of skin diseases, such as lupus vulgaris, using light therapy. Finsen's work illuminated the path for further research into the healing properties of light.

Low-Level Laser Therapy (LLLT) Emerges (1960s-1970s)

The 1960s marked a pivotal moment in the history of light therapy with the invention of the laser. Lasers, or Light Amplification by Stimulated Emission of Radiation, generated focused and intense beams of light. This innovation opened up new possibilities in medical treatment.

Around the same time, a serendipitous discovery by Endre Mester, a Hungarian physician, set the stage for the birth of Low-Level Laser Therapy (LLLT). Mester found that low-level laser light, initially believed to be harmless, stimulated hair growth in mice. This unexpected finding unveiled the potential of using low-level laser light for therapeutic purposes.

The Advent of Light-Emitting Diodes (LEDs) (1980s-1990s)

In the following decades, the development of light-emitting diodes (LEDs) became a pivotal advancement in light therapy. LEDs emitted specific wavelengths of light, including red and near-infrared, without the concentrated intensity of lasers. This made them safer and more versatile for a wide range of applications.

Scientific and Clinical Exploration (1990s-Present)
Throughout the 1990s and into the 21st century, researchers delved deeper into the therapeutic potential of red and near-infrared light. Studies began to explore the effects of
light on cellular function, tissue repair, and pain management. It was during this period that red light therapy gained recognition for its ability to accelerate wound healing and tissue regeneration.

NASA's Contribution (Early 2000s)
Red light therapy garnered widespread attention when NASA conducted studies on its potential benefits for plant growth in space. In a twist of fate, these studies unintentionally revealed its remarkable effects on

human biology. NASA found that red light therapy not only promoted plant growth but also accelerated wound healing and tissue repair in astronauts. This discovery piqued the interest of the medical community and sparked further research into the applications of red light therapy for human health.

Cosmetic and Wellness Industry Adoption (2000s-Present)

The 21st century witnessed the integration of red light therapy into the cosmetic and wellness industry. Spas, wellness centers, and clinics began to offer red light therapy treatments for a wide range of purposes, including skin rejuvenation, anti-aging, pain relief, and even weight loss. The accessibility of red light therapy expanded as more devices became available.

Scientific Validation (2000s-Present)

In recent years, red light therapy has undergone rigorous scientific scrutiny, leading to a substantial body of evidence supporting its effectiveness. Research has explored its benefits in diverse fields, including dermatology (for skin conditions and anti-aging), sports medicine (for muscle recovery and performance enhancement), and physical therapy (for pain relief and injury recovery). These studies have contributed to the growing acceptance of red light therapy within the medical community.

Diverse Applications and Home Use (Present)
Today, red light therapy finds application in a wide array of fields. In dermatology, it is used to address skin conditions, reduce the visible signs of aging, and promote overall skin health. In sports medicine, athletes rely on it for faster recovery and improved performance. Physical therapists use it to alleviate pain and enhance the healing of injuries. Moreover, the availability of consumer-grade red light therapy devices has democratized access to this treatment. Individuals can now incorporate red light therapy into their daily routines for a myriad of health and wellness benefits.

The Future of Red Light Therapy.
As research continues to unveil the remarkable potential of red light therapy, it is poised to evolve further and find new applications in healthcare and

wellness. With its non-invasive, safe, and scientifically supported approach, red light therapy is likely to continue illuminating the path to improved health and well-being in the years to come.

The history of red light therapy stands as a testament to human curiosity and innovation. From the pioneering work of early visionaries to the cutting-edge research of today, it exemplifies how science and technology can merge to create transformative solutions for human health and wellness.

The Science Behind Red Light Therapy :In-depth exploration of how red and near-infrared light affect the skin at a cellular level.

In the quest for radiant, youthful skin and improved overall well-being, the world of red light therapy emerges as a beacon of hope. But what exactly is the science behind this innovative therapeutic approach, and how does it work its magic on our skin and cells? Let's embark on a journey to illuminate the intricate science behind red light therapy.

The Spectrum of Healing Light

Before we delve into the inner workings of red light therapy, we must first grasp the concept of the electromagnetic spectrum—a vast expanse of energies, from high-energy X-rays to gentle radio waves. Within this spectrum, we find visible light, a mere sliver of the spectrum's breadth. Nestled within this tiny segment are the wavelengths that hold the promise of healing.

Red and Near-Infrared Light: The stars of red light therapy are the red and near-infrared wavelengths, typically ranging from approximately 620 to 1100 nanometers. These wavelengths are special; they possess unique properties that set them apart. They have the remarkable ability to penetrate the skin's surface, reaching deep into the tissues where the magic unfolds.

Cellular Energization: Unveiling the Mitochondria

To grasp the science behind red light therapy, we must venture into the inner sanctum of our cells, where a tiny yet potent organelle resides—the mitochondria. Often referred to as the cell's "powerhouse," mitochondria play a pivotal role in our bodies' energy production.

ATP: The Currency of Cellular Energy: At the heart of cellular energy lies adenosine triphosphate (ATP). It's the fuel that powers cellular functions, enabling them to carry out vital processes. Within the mitochondria, complex chemical reactions churn away, producing ATP.

The Photobiomodulation Phenomenon: The real enchantment of red light therapy, also known as photobiomodulation, hinges on the intricate dance between red and near-infrared light and the mitochondria. When these gentle wavelengths encounter our cells, they are absorbed by the mitochondria, initiating a cascade of biochemical reactions.

Stimulating ATP Production: This interaction stimulates the mitochondria to ramp up ATP production. It's akin to giving the cellular engines a boost, ensuring that cells have an abundance of energy to carry out their functions optimally.

A Collagen Revival: Red light therapy doesn't stop at cellular energy production; it has another captivating trick up its sleeve. These wavelengths have been shown to stimulate fibroblast cells to synthesize collagen—a crucial protein responsible for skin's elasticity and youthfulness. As we age, collagen production tends to decline, leading to the formation of wrinkles and fine lines. Red light therapy effectively nudges our bodies to rejuvenate collagen, promoting smoother, more youthful skin.

Reducing Inflammation: Inflammation is a common foe in the battle for healthy skin. Red light therapy has shown promise in reducing inflammation by modulating the production of inflammatory mediators. This anti-inflammatory effect can be particularly beneficial for individuals with conditions like acne or rosacea.

Enhancing Blood Flow: Proper blood circulation is essential for nourishing skin cells with oxygen and nutrients. Red light therapy has been demonstrated to enhance blood flow in the skin, ensuring that cells receive the sustenance they need to thrive.

The Practical Application: Understanding the science behind red light therapy is fascinating, but how is this knowledge applied in real life? Red light therapy devices, often in the form of panels, masks, or handheld devices, emit these precise wavelengths that penetrate the skin. When used as directed, they stimulate the desired cellular responses, fostering healthier, more youthful skin.

Safety and Minimal Heat: One of the remarkable aspects of red light therapy is its safety. Unlike some treatments that generate significant heat, red light therapy devices remain cool to the touch. There is minimal risk of burns or damage to the skin.

Non-Invasive and Painless: Red light therapy is non-invasive and painless, making it an attractive option for individuals seeking skincare solutions without the discomfort or downtime associated with surgical procedures.

As we unravel the science behind red light therapy, we uncover a world where gentle wavelengths of light hold the power to invigorate our cells, promote collagen revival, reduce inflammation, and enhance blood flow. This science-backed approach is a testament to the remarkable potential of harnessing the forces of nature to nurture radiant, youthful skin and overall well-being.

Benefits of Red Light Therapy for Skin: Discussing the various ways red light therapy can improve skin health, including reducing wrinkles, promoting collagen production, and addressing acne.

Radiant, youthful skin is a universal aspiration, and red light therapy emerges as a potent ally in this pursuit. This innovative therapeutic approach, bathed in gentle wavelengths of red and near-infrared light, unveils a treasure trove of benefits for skin health. Let's explore how red light therapy can transform your complexion by reducing wrinkles, promoting collagen production, and addressing acne.

Diminishing Wrinkles and Fine Lines

One of the most coveted promises of red light therapy is its ability to turn back the hands of time, reducing the visible signs of aging etched in the form of wrinkles and fine lines. The science behind this phenomenon is elegant in its simplicity. Red and near-infrared light, when absorbed by the skin's cells, particularly the fibroblasts, act as a gentle nudge to kickstart collagen production.

Collagen's Crucial Role: Collagen, the structural protein responsible for skin's elasticity and youthful firmness, tends to dwindle with age. The consequence? Skin begins to sag, and wrinkles make their unwelcome appearance. Red light therapy rekindles the collagen synthesis process, helping to rebuild the scaffolding of your skin.

A Smooth and Youthful Complexion: As collagen levels rise, you'll notice a transformation. Skin becomes firmer, plumper, and more resilient. Wrinkles and fine lines gradually fade into the background, replaced by a smoother, more youthful complexion. The results are subtle yet profound, like a masterpiece being meticulously restored.

Promoting Collagen Production: It's not just about replenishing existing collagen; red light therapy can also stimulate the production of new collagen. This dynamic duo—collagen revival and production—ensures that your skin is not only renewed but fortified against the relentless march of time.

Addressing the Acne Dilemma

Acne, a common skin woe that can afflict individuals of all ages, finds a formidable adversary in red light therapy. Unlike harsh chemical treatments, red light therapy offers a gentler, yet effective approach to managing acne.

Taming Inflammation: Acne often goes hand in hand with inflammation. Red light therapy, with its anti-inflammatory prowess, can help soothe the angry, red bumps and pustules that accompany acne outbreaks. It does so by modulating the production of inflammatory mediators, pacifying the skin's fiery response.

Healing and Recovery: Red light therapy supports the skin's natural healing processes. It can accelerate the resolution of blemishes, minimize scarring, and promote the recovery of healthy skin. It's like sending in a skilled craftsman to repair the damage caused by acne, ensuring minimal traces are left behind.

Balancing Sebum Production: Acne can be exacerbated by overactive sebaceous glands, leading to excess oil production. Red light therapy can help restore balance by regulating sebum production. This means fewer clogged pores and a reduced likelihood of new breakouts.

A Multifaceted Approach to Skin Health

In the world of skin care, red light therapy stands as a multifaceted tool. It doesn't simply mask imperfections; it addresses them at their roots. Whether you're battling wrinkles, seeking to rejuvenate your complexion, or waging war against acne, red light therapy's gentle yet powerful wavelengths offer a science-backed path to radiant skin. By promoting collagen production, reducing inflammation, and supporting the skin's natural healing processes, red light therapy unlocks the door to a healthier, more youthful complexion.

Enhancing Skin Health Holistically

The benefits of red light therapy extend beyond its targeted effects on wrinkles, collagen, and acne. It encompasses a holistic approach to skin health that touches upon various aspects of your complexion:

Reduction in Redness and Rosacea: Individuals with skin conditions like rosacea often contend with persistent redness and flushing. Red light therapy can help mitigate these symptoms by calming the skin's reactivity and reducing redness over time.

Improved Skin Texture: Beyond the visual improvements, many individuals report that their skin feels smoother and more refined after red light therapy sessions. This enhanced texture can be attributed to the combination of collagen regeneration and improved circulation.

Minimization of Scars: Whether you have scars from acne, injuries, or surgical procedures, red light therapy may play a role in minimizing their appearance. By promoting tissue repair and collagen synthesis, it supports the gradual fading of scars.

Hydration and Radiance: Skin health is closely tied to hydration, and red light therapy may contribute to improved skin hydration. Well-hydrated skin appears more radiant and vibrant, further enhancing your complexion.

Anti-Aging Beyond the Surface: Red light therapy doesn't just focus on the outermost layer of skin; it works its magic deep within. This approach ensures that your skin not only looks youthful but also functions optimally, maintaining its resilience and vitality over time.

Customizing Your Red Light Therapy Journey

When embarking on your red light therapy journey, it's important to customize your approach to your specific skin goals and needs. The duration and frequency of sessions, as well as the choice of red or near-infrared wavelengths, can be tailored to address your unique concerns. Some individuals opt for professional red light therapy treatments, while others prefer at-home devices for ongoing skincare maintenance.

In conclusion, red light therapy is more than a cosmetic remedy; it's a science-backed strategy for enhancing skin health from the inside out. By reducing wrinkles, promoting collagen production, and addressing acne, it addresses common skin concerns while also contributing to a holistic and radiant complexion. As you embark on your own journey to healthier, more youthful skin, consider the multifaceted benefits that red light therapy has to offer.

Choosing the Right Red Light Therapy Device: Guidance on selecting the appropriate device for at-home or professional use.

Embarking on your journey with red light therapy is an exciting step towards improving your skin health and overall well-being. Whether you're considering using red light therapy at home or seeking professional treatments, selecting the right device is crucial. Let's delve into the key factors to consider when choosing the perfect red light therapy device for your needs.

1. **Device Type: Red light therapy devices come in various forms, each with its own advantages:

- **Panel or Panel Array**: These large devices emit light over a broad area, making them suitable for full-body treatments. They are often used in professional settings but are also available for home use.

- **Mask**: Red light therapy masks are designed to treat the face and neck. They are convenient for at-home use and are particularly popular for targeting facial skin concerns.

- **Handheld Devices**: These compact devices are easy to maneuver and are suitable for both targeted and full-body treatments. They are a versatile option for home use.

- **Combination Devices**: Some devices offer a combination of red light therapy with other technologies, such as blue light for acne treatment or infrared for deep tissue penetration. Consider your specific goals when choosing a device.

2. **Wavelengths: Red light therapy devices typically emit light in the red and near-infrared spectrum. Ensure that the device you choose offers the specific wavelengths that align with your intended benefits. Common wavelengths for skin-related purposes range from around 620 to 850 nanometers.

3. **Intensity and Power: The power or intensity of the device's light output is an important consideration. Professional-grade devices tend to have higher power levels, while at-home devices vary in intensity. Consider your skin goals and sensitivity when selecting the appropriate power level.

4. **Treatment Area: Determine the size of the treatment area you wish to cover. Some devices are designed for small, targeted areas like the face, while others can accommodate larger areas or even the entire body.

5. **Ease of Use: Consider the ease of use and convenience of the device. Look for features such as timers, adjustable intensity settings, and user-friendly controls.

6. **Safety Features: Ensure that the device has safety features such as eye protection (for devices that emit visible light) and automatic shut-off timers to prevent overuse.

7. **Quality and Brand: Research reputable brands and read reviews to ensure the quality and reliability of the device. Look for devices that have been tested and certified for safety and effectiveness.

8. **Budget: Set a budget that aligns with your financial constraints. Red light therapy devices come in a wide price range, so there are options available for various budgets.

9. **Professional vs. Home Use: Decide whether you prefer professional treatments or the convenience of at-home use. Professional treatments are typically administered by trained practitioners and may involve more powerful devices. At-home devices offer convenience and can be used on your schedule.

10. **Consultation: If you have specific skin concerns or medical conditions, it's advisable to consult with a healthcare professional or dermatologist before selecting a red light therapy device. They can provide guidance based on your individual needs.

Remember that consistency is key when it comes to red light therapy, so choose a device that aligns with your lifestyle and treatment goals. Whether you opt for a mask, panel, handheld device, or combination device, the right choice will empower you to embark on your red light therapy journey with confidence and the potential for transformative results.

How to Use Red Light Therapy Safely: Information on safe and effective usage, including session duration and frequency.

Red light therapy holds great promise for enhancing skin health and overall well-being. To unlock its full potential, it's essential to use this therapy safely and effectively. Here's a comprehensive guide on how to use red light therapy safely, including session duration and frequency:

1. **Consultation: Before beginning any red light therapy regimen, consider consulting with a healthcare professional or dermatologist, especially if you have specific skin concerns or underlying medical conditions. They can provide tailored recommendations and ensure the therapy aligns with your needs.

2. **Device Safety: Ensure that your red light therapy device is certified for safety and effectiveness. Read the user manual thoroughly to understand its operation and safety features, such as timers and eye protection, if applicable.

3. **Eye Protection: Some red light therapy devices emit visible light that can be harmful to the eyes. If your device emits visible light, always use the provided eye protection goggles during sessions to shield your eyes.

4. **Clean, Dry Skin: Before using the device, ensure that your skin is clean and dry. Remove any makeup, lotions, or oils from the treatment area to maximize light penetration.

5. **Treatment Area: Identify the area of your body you wish to treat. Red light therapy can be used on the face, neck, body, or specific targeted areas, depending on your goals.

6. **Distance: Follow the manufacturer's recommendations regarding the distance between the device and your skin. Maintaining the correct distance ensures that you receive the intended light intensity.

7. **Session Duration: Session duration can vary based on the device's power and your goals. In general, sessions can range from a few minutes to 20-30 minutes. Start with shorter sessions and gradually increase the duration as your skin becomes accustomed to the therapy.

8. **Frequency: The frequency of red light therapy sessions depends on your goals and the device's specifications. For many skin-related concerns, such as reducing wrinkles or promoting collagen production, using the device 3-5 times per week is common. However, consult the device's manual and your healthcare professional for personalized recommendations.

9. **Consistency: Consistency is key to seeing results with red light therapy. Stick to a regular schedule that aligns with your goals. Skipping sessions or using the device irregularly may limit its effectiveness.

10. **Hydration: Maintain proper hydration by drinking water before and after each session. Well-hydrated skin can respond more effectively to red light therapy.

11. **Skin Sensation: During sessions, you may feel a gentle warming sensation on your skin. This is normal and is a sign that the therapy is working. However, if you experience discomfort or excessive heat, stop the session immediately.

12. **Monitor Progress: Keep a record of your sessions and track your progress over time. Take photos to document changes in your skin's appearance.

13. **Caution with Medications: If you are taking medications that increase photosensitivity, such as certain antibiotics or topical treatments, consult with your healthcare provider before starting red light therapy.

14. **Skin Protection: Following sessions, protect your skin from excessive sun exposure. Red light therapy can make your skin more sensitive to UV rays, so apply sunscreen or protective clothing if you plan to be outdoors.

15. **Maintenance: Follow the manufacturer's guidelines for maintaining your device. Keep it clean and in good working condition.

By adhering to these safe practices and guidelines, you can harness the potential of red light therapy to promote radiant skin while minimizing any potential risks or adverse effects. If you ever have concerns or questions, don't hesitate to seek guidance from a healthcare professional or the device manufacturer

Combining Red Light Therapy with Skincare: Tips on incorporating red light therapy into your skincare routine and session

Elevating your skincare routine with the addition of red light therapy can be a transformative experience. This dynamic duo offers the potential for healthier, more radiant skin. Here are some tips on how to seamlessly incorporate red light therapy into your skincare routine and maximize its effectiveness:

1. **Cleanse Your Canvas: Always start with a clean slate. Gently cleanse your face or the treatment area to remove makeup, dirt, and excess oils. Clean skin allows red and near-infrared light to penetrate more effectively.

2. **Choose Appropriate Skincare Products: While red light therapy can work wonders on its own, you can enhance its effects by using complementary skincare products. Look for products that are rich in antioxidants, hyaluronic acid, and peptides, which can support skin hydration, repair, and collagen production.

3. **Apply Skincare Products Before Red Light Therapy: If you're combining red light therapy with skincare products, apply them before your therapy session. This allows the active ingredients in your products to better penetrate the skin during the session.

4. **Moisturize: After your red light therapy session, apply a hydrating and nourishing moisturizer to lock in the benefits. This can help soothe the skin and keep it well-hydrated.

5. **Be Consistent: Incorporate red light therapy into your skincare routine consistently. Consistency is key to seeing long-term improvements in your skin's health and appearance.

6. **Understand Wavelengths: Different wavelengths of red and near-infrared light can target specific skin concerns. Understand which wavelengths your device emits and how they align with your skincare goals.

7. **Session Duration: Pay attention to session duration. While shorter sessions are typically safe, extended exposure may not always be beneficial. Follow the recommended session duration for your specific device and goals.

8. **Combine with Serums: Consider using serums that contain ingredients like vitamin C, retinol, or peptides before red light therapy. These can work synergistically with the therapy to promote collagen production and skin rejuvenation.

9. **Post-Treatment Care: After your session, avoid applying harsh or irritating skincare products immediately. Allow your skin to recover and then resume your regular skincare routine.

10. **Sun Protection: Red light therapy can make your skin more sensitive to UV rays. As part of your skincare routine, always apply sunscreen when going outside to protect your skin from sun damage.

11. **Adjust to Your Skin Goals: Tailor your red light therapy sessions and skincare products to your specific skin goals. Whether it's reducing wrinkles, improving skin texture, or addressing acne, align your routine with your desired outcomes.

12. **Professional Advice: If you have complex skin concerns or are unsure how to combine red light therapy with your skincare routine, consult a dermatologist or skin care professional. They can provide personalized recommendations.

13. **Monitor Progress: Keep track of your skin's progress over time. Take photos to document changes in texture, tone, and overall appearance.

14. **Hydrate Adequately: Drinking enough water is essential for skin health. Proper hydration can complement the effects of red light therapy, helping your skin appear more radiant and plump.

15. **Be Patient: Skincare results often take time, and the same applies to red light therapy. Be patient and consistent with your routine. It may take several weeks to months to see significant improvements, so stay committed.

16. **Rotate Your Skincare Products: While consistency is crucial, periodically rotating skincare products can prevent your skin from becoming too accustomed to a single regimen. Consult with a skincare professional for guidance on when and how to switch products.

17. **Tailor Your Routine to Time of Day: Some individuals prefer to use red light therapy in the morning, while others choose evening sessions. Tailor your skincare routine accordingly, considering factors like sun exposure and product compatibility.

18. **Consider Targeted Treatments: If you have specific skincare concerns, consider using targeted treatments alongside red light therapy. For instance, if you're combating acne, incorporate acne-fighting products into your routine.

19. **Detoxify Your Skin: Regularly exfoliate your skin to remove dead skin cells and improve light penetration during red light therapy sessions. However, be gentle to avoid over-exfoliation.

20. **Embrace a Holistic Approach: Remember that skincare isn't just about external treatments. A balanced diet, exercise, and stress management also play vital roles in skin health. Adopting a holistic approach can complement the benefits of red light therapy.

21. **Take Breaks: While consistency is crucial, it's also beneficial to allow your skin to breathe. Consider taking short breaks from red light therapy to assess your skin's progress and ensure you're not overusing the treatment.

22. **Professional Guidance: If you're new to red light therapy or have complex skin concerns, consider seeking professional guidance. A dermatologist or licensed skin care professional can provide expert advice and recommend suitable products and treatments.

23. **Skin Patch Testing: When introducing new skincare products alongside red light therapy, perform a patch test on a small area of your skin to ensure you don't experience adverse reactions.

24. **Stay Informed: Stay updated on the latest skincare trends, ingredients, and innovations. The skincare industry is constantly evolving, and being informed can help you make informed choices.

25. **Listen to Your Skin: Your skin is unique, and what works for one person may not work for another. Pay attention to how your skin responds to red light therapy and skincare products, and adjust your routine accordingly.

By integrating these tips into your skincare routine, you can create a comprehensive and personalized approach to achieve your desired skin goals. Red light therapy, when combined with thoughtful skin care practices, can be a powerful tool for nurturing radiant and healthy skin.

Skin Conditions and Red Light Therapy: Detailed guidance on how red light therapy can help specific skin conditions such as eczema, psoriasis, and rosacea.

Red light therapy isn't just a one-size-fits-all solution; it's a versatile approach that can be tailored to address specific skin conditions. Here's a comprehensive guide on how red light therapy can help alleviate common skin issues like eczema, psoriasis, and rosacea:

1. **Eczema:

   - **Understanding Eczema**: Eczema, also known as atopic dermatitis, is characterized by red, itchy, and inflamed skin. It's often a chronic condition with periods of flare-ups and remission.

   - **How Red Light Therapy Helps**:

- **Anti-Inflammatory Effects**: Red light therapy's anti-inflammatory properties can help reduce redness and swelling associated with eczema.

- **Improved Healing**: By stimulating the skin's natural healing processes, red light therapy can promote faster recovery from eczema flare-ups and reduce the risk of infection.

- **Itch Relief**: Many eczema sufferers experience intense itching. Red light therapy may help alleviate itching sensations, providing relief.

- **Application**: Use red light therapy as part of your skincare routine, focusing on affected areas. Regular sessions during flare-ups and maintenance sessions during remission can be beneficial.

2. **Psoriasis:

- **Understanding Psoriasis**: Psoriasis is characterized by raised, scaly, and often itchy patches of skin. It's an autoimmune condition that can vary in severity.

- **How Red Light Therapy Helps**:

  - **Slowing Cell Growth**: Red light therapy may slow down the rapid growth of skin cells, a hallmark of psoriasis. This can help reduce the thickness and scaling of psoriatic plaques.

    - **Anti-Inflammatory Properties**: Like with eczema, red light therapy's anti-inflammatory effects can help reduce redness and inflammation in psoriasis-affected areas.

- **Application**: Use red light therapy specifically on psoriasis-affected areas. The frequency and duration of sessions can vary based on the severity of your condition.

3. **Rosacea:

  - **Understanding Rosacea**: Rosacea is a chronic skin condition that leads to facial redness, visible blood vessels, and sometimes pimple-like bumps. It often has triggers like heat, alcohol, or spicy foods.

  - **How Red Light Therapy Helps**:

- **Reducing Redness**: Red light therapy can target and reduce the redness associated with rosacea.

- **Strengthening Blood Vessels**: Some studies suggest that red light therapy may help strengthen blood vessels, potentially reducing their visibility on the skin.

- **Application**: Incorporate red light therapy into your skincare routine, focusing on rosacea-prone areas like the cheeks and nose. Regular sessions can help manage symptoms and maintain clearer skin.

4. **General Tips for Skin Conditions:

- **Consultation**: Before starting red light therapy for a skin condition, consult with a dermatologist or healthcare professional for personalized advice.

- **Consistency**: Consistency is key. Develop a regular schedule for red light therapy sessions, and be patient with the process, as improvements may take time.

- **Complementary Products**: Consider using skincare products specifically formulated for your skin condition in conjunction with red light therapy. Consult with a dermatologist for product recommendations.

- **Sun Protection**: Skin conditions can make your skin more sensitive to sunlight. Always apply sunscreen when going outdoors to protect your skin.

- **Monitor Progress**: Keep track of your skin's progress over time. Document changes in redness, itching, or scaling to gauge the effectiveness of red light therapy.

Red light therapy offers a promising avenue for managing and improving the symptoms of skin conditions like eczema, psoriasis, and rosacea. By understanding your specific condition, adhering to a consistent treatment plan, and consulting with professionals, you can harness the potential of red light therapy to nurture healthier, more comfortable skin.

Anti-Aging Strategies: A comprehensive look at how red light therapy can contribute to a youthful complexion and reduce the signs of aging.

Aging is a natural process, but with the emergence of advanced skin care techniques, we have the power to age gracefully. Red light therapy stands at the forefront of these techniques, offering a comprehensive approach to a youthful complexion. Let's delve into how red light therapy can be a key component of your anti-aging strategy:

1. **Collagen Production and Wrinkle Reduction:

  - **Collagen, the Youth Elixir**: Collagen is a protein that provides structure to your skin, keeping it firm and smooth. As we age, collagen production naturally declines, leading to the formation of wrinkles and fine lines.

  - **Red Light Therapy's Role**:
    - **Stimulating Collagen Synthesis**: Red light therapy has been shown to stimulate fibroblast cells,

which are responsible for collagen production. This stimulation encourages the synthesis of new collagen, leading to improved skin elasticity and reduced wrinkles.

2. **Cellular Energy Boost:

   - **Cellular Powerhouses**: Within our cells, mitochondria are the powerhouses responsible for energy production. With age, mitochondrial function can decline, impacting the overall health and appearance of the skin.

  - **Red Light Therapy's Role**:
   - **Enhancing ATP Production**: Red light therapy interacts with mitochondria, increasing the production of adenosine triphosphate (ATP), the primary source of cellular energy. This boost in energy can enhance cellular function, promoting healthier and more youthful skin.

3. **Reduction in Inflammation:

- **Inflammation and Aging**: Chronic inflammation is a common contributor to premature aging. It can lead to skin redness, irritation, and the breakdown of collagen and elastin fibers.

  - **Red Light Therapy's Role**:
    - **Anti-Inflammatory Effects**: Red light therapy exhibits anti-inflammatory properties, helping to reduce skin inflammation. This can lead to a calmer, more even-toned complexion.

4. **Enhanced Blood Circulation:

  - **Blood Flow for Vitality**: Proper blood circulation is crucial for delivering oxygen and nutrients to skin cells. As we age, blood circulation can become less efficient.

  - **Red Light Therapy's Role**:
    - **Improved Blood Flow**: Red light therapy has been shown to enhance blood circulation in the skin. This ensures that skin cells receive the nourishment they need to thrive, promoting a vibrant complexion.

5. **Improved Skin Texture and Tone:

- **Texture Matters**: Uneven skin texture and tone are common signs of aging. These issues can manifest as rough patches, age spots, or discoloration.

- **Red Light Therapy's Role**:
  - **Enhanced Cellular Turnover**: Red light therapy can support the skin's natural processes of cellular turnover, helping to shed dead skin cells and promote a smoother, more even skin tone.

6. **Pain-Free and Non-Invasive:

- **Gentle Approach**: Unlike some anti-aging treatments that may be invasive or painful, red light therapy is non-invasive and pain-free. It offers an attractive alternative for those seeking anti-aging solutions without discomfort.

7. **Home Use Convenience:

- **At-Home Devices**: Red light therapy devices designed for home use provide the convenience of integrating anti-aging treatments into your daily routine. This accessibility allows for consistent use, which is key to achieving lasting results.

8. **Complementary to Other Treatments:

- **Combination Potential**: Red light therapy can complement other anti-aging treatments, such as topical serums or cosmetic procedures. It enhances the overall efficacy of your anti-aging strategy.

9. **Preventative Approach:

- **Starting Early**: While red light therapy is effective for addressing existing signs of aging, it can also be used preventatively. Starting a red light therapy routine in your younger years can help maintain youthful skin as you age.

10. **Personalized Approach:

- **Tailored to Your Needs**: Red light therapy is versatile and can be tailored to your specific skin concerns and goals. Whether you're targeting wrinkles, uneven skin tone, or overall skin health, you can customize your approach.

Red light therapy shines as a beacon of hope for those seeking effective and holistic anti-aging solutions. Its ability to stimulate collagen production, enhance cellular energy, reduce inflammation, and improve blood circulation makes it a valuable addition to your skincare regimen. As you embark on your journey toward a more youthful complexion, consider the radiant possibilities that red light therapy offers.

Case Studies and Success Stories: Real-life examples of individuals who have experienced positive results with red light therapy.

- Lisa's Journey to Eczema Relief
- **Background**: Lisa, a 28-year-old nurse, had struggled with eczema since childhood. Her eczema primarily affected her hands and wrists, causing intense itching, redness, and painful flare-ups.

- **Red Light Therapy Journey**: Lisa had tried numerous creams and ointments to manage her eczema, but they provided only temporary relief. She decided to explore alternative treatments and came across red light therapy. Lisa purchased a handheld red light therapy device designed for home use and began using it for 10-minute sessions daily.

- **Results**: Over a few weeks, Lisa noticed a significant improvement in her eczema symptoms. The red light therapy sessions helped reduce the itching and inflammation on her hands. The skin on her wrists, which had been prone to painful cracks during eczema flare-ups, started to heal more rapidly. Lisa's overall skin condition became more manageable, and she experienced fewer severe flare-ups.

Lisa's journey with red light therapy not only provided her with relief from the discomfort of eczema but also improved her quality of life. It allowed her to perform her nursing duties with greater comfort and confidence, demonstrating how this non-invasive therapy can make a meaningful difference in the lives of individuals with chronic skin conditions.

The proof of any skincare or anti-aging treatment lies in the real-life experiences of individuals who have witnessed transformative results.

- Jane's Wrinkle Reversal

*Background**: Jane, a 50-year-old marketing executive, had begun to notice the subtle yet persistent signs of aging on her face, including fine lines and wrinkles.

- **Red Light Therapy Journey**: Jane decided to incorporate red light therapy into her skincare routine. She used a red light therapy device at home for 20-minute sessions, three times a week.

- **Results**: Over several months, Jane experienced a noticeable reduction in the appearance of fine lines and wrinkles. Her skin felt firmer and more radiant. Jane's success with red light therapy boosted her confidence and helped her maintain a youthful complexion.

- Mike's Rosacea Relief
Background: Mike, a 38-year-old teacher, had struggled with rosacea for years. He experienced frequent redness and visible blood vessels on his cheeks and nose.

- **Red Light Therapy Journey**: Mike consulted with a dermatologist who recommended red light therapy as a part of his rosacea management plan. He received in-office red light therapy treatments twice a week for several weeks.

- **Results**: Mike's rosacea symptoms significantly improved. The redness on his face diminished, and the visible blood vessels became less pronounced. He experienced fewer flare-ups, and his skin regained a healthier appearance.

- Sarah's Acne Recovery

Background: Sarah, a 25-year-old student, had been battling acne since her teenage years. She had tried various topical treatments and antibiotics without achieving clear skin.

- **Red Light Therapy Journey**: Sarah discovered the potential of red light therapy for acne management. She began using a red light therapy mask at home for 15-minute sessions, five times a week.

- **Results**: Over a few months, Sarah's acne gradually improved. Her breakouts became less frequent and less severe. The red light therapy helped reduce inflammation and allowed her skin to heal more effectively.

- David's Psoriasis Progress

*Background**: David, a 45-year-old accountant, had lived with psoriasis for over a decade. He had tried various treatments, including topical corticosteroids, with limited success.

- **Red Light Therapy Journey**: David's dermatologist recommended red light therapy as an additional treatment. He received in-office red light therapy sessions twice a week for several months.

- **Results**: David's psoriasis plaques became less thick and scaly. The red light therapy helped slow down the rapid cell turnover characteristic of psoriasis. He experienced a significant reduction in the discomfort associated with psoriasis.

These case studies and success stories offer a glimpse into the tangible benefits that individuals have achieved through red light therapy. While results may vary from person to person, these real-life examples highlight the versatility and effectiveness of red light therapy in addressing a wide range of skin concerns. Whether it's wrinkle reduction, rosacea relief, acne management, or psoriasis progress, red light therapy has shown its potential to transform lives and restore confidence in one's skin.

Diet and Lifestyle for Radiant Skin**: Exploring the role of nutrition, hydration, and healthy habits in maintaining skin health alongside red light therapy.

While red light therapy can work wonders for your skin, it's important to remember that skincare is a holistic journey. What you eat, how you hydrate, and your lifestyle choices can significantly impact your skin's health and radiance. Let's explore the essential aspects of diet and lifestyle that can complement your red light therapy regimen:

1. **Nutrition for Skin Health:

   - **Hydration**: Start with the basics—hydration. Drinking plenty of water helps maintain skin moisture and supports overall skin health. Adequate hydration ensures that your skin functions optimally.

   - **Antioxidants**: Incorporate foods rich in antioxidants into your diet. These include fruits like berries, citrus, and kiwi, as well as vegetables like spinach, kale, and carrots. Antioxidants help protect your skin from free radical damage, which can accelerate the aging process.

- **Healthy Fats**: Omega-3 fatty acids found in fatty fish, flaxseeds, and walnuts can help keep your skin supple and hydrated. These fats are essential for maintaining the skin's lipid barrier.

- **Protein**: Protein sources like lean meats, poultry, beans, and tofu provide the amino acids needed for collagen production, supporting skin firmness.

- **Vitamins and Minerals**: Ensure your diet includes vitamins and minerals that promote skin health, such as vitamin C (found in citrus fruits and broccoli), vitamin E (found in nuts and seeds), and zinc (found in beans and whole grains).

2. **Healthy Habits for Radiant Skin:

- **Regular Exercise**: Physical activity enhances blood circulation, delivering oxygen and nutrients to skin cells. It also helps remove toxins through sweat, promoting clearer skin.

- **Adequate Sleep**: Quality sleep is essential for skin repair and regeneration. Aim for 7-9 hours of restful sleep each night to allow your skin to rejuvenate.

- **Stress Management**: Chronic stress can lead to skin issues like breakouts and exacerbate conditions like eczema and psoriasis. Practicing stress management techniques, such as meditation or yoga, can benefit your skin.

- **Sun Protection**: Protect your skin from UV damage by wearing sunscreen and protective clothing when exposed to the sun. UV rays can accelerate skin aging and increase the risk of skin cancer.

3. **Red Light Therapy Synergy:

- **Consistency**: Just as with your diet and lifestyle choices, consistency with red light therapy sessions is crucial for optimal results. Follow a regular schedule to maximize the benefits.

- **Preparation**: Ensure your skin is clean and free from makeup or skincare products before each red light therapy session. This allows for better light penetration.

- **Post-Session Care**: After a red light therapy session, apply a hydrating moisturizer to lock in the benefits and soothe your skin.

- **Sunscreen**: Be mindful of sun exposure after red light therapy sessions. Red light therapy can make your skin more sensitive to UV rays, so apply sunscreen as needed.

4. **Personalized Approach:

- **Unique Needs**: Remember that everyone's skin is unique. What works for one person may not work for another. Tailor your diet, lifestyle, and red light therapy routine to your specific skin concerns and goals.

5. **Hydrate Adequately: Drinking enough water is essential for skin health. Proper hydration can complement the effects of red light therapy, helping your skin appear more radiant and plump.

6. **Be Patient: Skincare results often take time, and the same applies to red light therapy. Be patient and consistent with your routine. It may take several weeks to months to see significant improvements, so stay committed.

7. **Rotate Your Skincare Products: While consistency is crucial, periodically rotating skincare products can prevent your skin from becoming too accustomed to a single regimen. Consult with a skincare professional for guidance on when and how to switch products.

8. **Tailor Your Routine to Time of Day: Some individuals prefer to use red light therapy in the morning, while others choose evening sessions. Tailor your skincare routine accordingly, considering factors like sun exposure and product compatibility.

9. **Consider Targeted Treatments: If you have specific skincare concerns, consider using targeted treatments alongside red light therapy. For instance, if you're combating acne, incorporate acne-fighting products into your routine.

10. **Detoxify Your Skin: Regularly exfoliate your skin to remove dead skin cells and improve light penetration during red light therapy sessions. However, be gentle to avoid over-exfoliation.

11. **Embrace a Holistic Approach: Remember that skincare isn't just about external treatments. A balanced diet, exercise, and stress management also play vital roles in skin health. Adopting a holistic approach can complement the benefits of red light therapy.

12. **Take Breaks: While consistency is crucial, it's also beneficial to allow your skin to breathe. Consider taking short breaks from red light therapy to assess your skin's progress and ensure you're not overusing the treatment.

13. **Professional Guidance: If you're new to red light therapy or have complex skin concerns, consider seeking professional guidance. A dermatologist or licensed skin care professional can provide expert advice and recommend suitable products and treatments.

14. **Skin Patch Testing: When introducing new skincare products alongside red light therapy, perform a patch test on a small area of your skin to ensure you don't experience adverse reactions.

15. **Stay Informed: Stay updated on the latest skincare trends, ingredients, and innovations. The skincare industry is constantly evolving, and being informed can help you make informed choices.

16. **Listen to Your Skin: Your skin is unique, and what works for one person may not work for another. Pay attention to how your skin responds to red light therapy and skincare products, and adjust your routine according

By combining the power of red light therapy with a balanced diet and a healthy lifestyle, you can create a comprehensive approach to radiant skin.

Complementary Skincare Products: Recommendations for skincare products and routines that work well with red light therapy.

Pairing red light therapy with the right skincare products can enhance the overall effectiveness of your skincare routine. Here are some recommendations for skincare products and routines that complement red light therapy:

1. **Gentle Cleanser:

   - **Why**: A gentle cleanser is essential to remove makeup, dirt, and impurities from your skin before a red light therapy session. Clean skin allows for better light penetration.

   - **Recommendation**: Look for a sulfate-free, hydrating cleanser that won't strip your skin's natural oils.

2. **Topical Antioxidants:

- **Why**: Antioxidants like vitamin C can help protect your skin from free radical damage and complement the anti-aging effects of red light therapy.

- **Recommendation**: Consider a vitamin C serum or cream to apply after your red light therapy session.

3. **Hyaluronic Acid Serum:

- **Why**: Hyaluronic acid is a hydrating powerhouse that can lock in moisture and support skin health.

- **Recommendation**: Apply a hyaluronic acid serum post-red light therapy to boost skin hydration.

4. **Retinol (Vitamin A):

- **Why**: Retinol is known for its ability to stimulate collagen production and promote skin renewal.

- **Recommendation**: Use a retinol product as part of your nighttime skincare routine, making sure it doesn't interfere with your red light therapy sessions.

5. **SPF Sunscreen:

- **Why**: After red light therapy, your skin may be more sensitive to UV rays. Sunscreen is crucial to protect your skin from sun damage.

- **Recommendation**: Opt for a broad-spectrum SPF 30 or higher sunscreen and apply it daily, especially if you're going outside.

6. **Moisturizer:

- **Why**: A good moisturizer helps keep your skin hydrated and seals in the benefits of red light therapy.

- **Recommendation**: Choose a moisturizer suitable for your skin type, whether it's dry, oily, or combination.

7. **Exfoliating Product:

- **Why**: Periodic exfoliation removes dead skin cells, ensuring that red light therapy penetrates effectively.

   - **Recommendation**: Use a gentle exfoliant (physical or chemical) as needed, but avoid over-exfoliating.

8. **Eye Cream:

   - **Why**: The delicate skin around the eyes may benefit from targeted treatments to address concerns like fine lines and puffiness.

   - **Recommendation**: Choose an eye cream that addresses your specific concerns, such as dark circles or wrinkles.

9. **Hydrating Mask:

   - **Why**: A hydrating mask can provide an extra boost of moisture and relaxation to your skincare routine.

- **Recommendation**: Use a hydrating mask once a week or as needed for a spa-like treat.

10. **Customization:

- **Why**: Your skincare needs are unique. Consult with a dermatologist or skin care professional to customize your product selection based on your skin type and concerns.

Skincare Routine with Red Light Therapy:

Here's a sample skincare routine that incorporates red light therapy:

Morning:

1. **Cleanser**: Start your day with a gentle cleanser to refresh your skin.

2. **Antioxidant Serum**: Apply a vitamin C serum to protect your skin from environmental damage.

3. **Sunscreen**: Finish with a broad-spectrum sunscreen to shield your skin from UV rays.

Evening:

1. **Cleanser**: Use a gentle cleanser to remove makeup and impurities.

2. **Red Light Therapy**: Follow the manufacturer's instructions for your red light therapy session.

3. **Retinol (if used)**: Apply retinol as part of your anti-aging routine, if recommended by your dermatologist.

4. **Hydrating Serum**: Use a hyaluronic acid serum to lock in moisture.

5. **Eye Cream**: Apply an eye cream to address specific eye area concerns.

6. **Moisturizer**: Finish with a moisturizer suitable for your skin type.

Weekly:

1. **Exfoliation**: Include exfoliation in your routine as needed, such as 1-2 times per week.

2. **Hydrating Mask**: Treat yourself to a hydrating mask once a week for an extra moisture boost.
Additional Skincare Tips and Considerations with Red Light Therapy:

11. **Patch Testing**: Whenever introducing new skincare products into your routine, especially if you have sensitive skin, perform a patch test on a small area to check for adverse reactions before applying them to your face or body.

12. **Professional Consultation: If you have specific skin concerns or conditions, consider consulting a dermatologist or skincare professional. They can provide personalized recommendations and treatments tailored to your needs.

13. **Product Shelf Life: Be mindful of the shelf life of your skincare products. Using expired products can be ineffective or even harmful to your skin.

14. **Avoid Overuse: While it's important to be consistent with your skincare routine, avoid overusing products or treatments. Over Exfoliating or using potent active ingredients too frequently can lead to skin irritation.

15. **Stay Informed: Stay updated on skincare trends, ingredients, and research. The skincare industry evolves, and new innovations can offer improved solutions for your skin concerns.

16. **Mindful Makeup Removal: If you wear makeup, ensure thorough makeup removal before red light therapy sessions. Makeup residue can block light penetration.

17. **Consistency Is Key: Stick to your skincare routine and red light therapy schedule to see the best results. The cumulative effects of these practices can lead to significant improvements over time.

18. **Adjust for Seasonal Changes: Your skincare needs may vary with changing seasons. Adapt your routine to account for differences in humidity, temperature, and sun exposure.

19. **Holistic Wellness: Remember that skincare isn't just about products—it's about holistic wellness. Maintain a balanced diet, manage stress, get regular exercise, and prioritize sleep for overall skin health.

20. **Share with Professionals: If you undergo professional skincare treatments or cosmetic procedures, inform your healthcare providers about your red light therapy routine. They can adjust their recommendations accordingly.

21. **Personalized Regimen: Ultimately, your skincare regimen should be tailored to your skin type, concerns, and goals. What works for one person may not work for another, so be open to customization.

By incorporating these additional skincare considerations into your routine alongside red light therapy, you can ensure a comprehensive and personalized approach to achieving your skincare goals. Whether your focus is anti-aging, acne management, or general skin health, these tips can help you make the most of your skincare journey.

Professional Red Light Therapy Treatments: Information on seeking professional red light therapy treatments and what to expect during a session

While many individuals opt for at-home red light therapy devices, seeking professional red light therapy treatments can provide a different level of care and expertise. Here's what you need to know about professional red light therapy sessions and what to expect during the process:

Why Choose Professional Red Light Therapy:

1. **Expertise**: Professionals, such as dermatologists or licensed aestheticians, have in-depth knowledge of skin conditions and can tailor red light therapy to your specific needs.

2. **Advanced Devices**: Professional settings often feature high-quality, medical-grade red light therapy devices with precise wavelength control.

3. **Optimal Results**: Professional treatments can yield faster and more dramatic results, especially for complex skin concerns.

What to Expect During a Professional Red Light Therapy Session:

1. **Consultation**: Your first session typically begins with a consultation. You'll discuss your skin concerns, goals, and any medical history. This information helps the professional create a personalized treatment plan.

2. **Skin Assessment**: The professional may assess your skin's condition, identifying areas of concern and determining the appropriate wavelength and intensity settings for your treatment.

3. **Preparation**: You'll be asked to cleanse your skin thoroughly before the session to remove makeup, skincare products, and oils. Clean skin allows the red light to penetrate more effectively.

4. **Protection**: You may wear protective eyewear to shield your eyes from the bright light. The professional will ensure your eyes are adequately protected.

5. **Session Duration**: Red light therapy sessions in a professional setting typically last 15 to 30 minutes, depending on your treatment plan and the specific device used.

6. **Application**: The professional will position the red light therapy device at the appropriate distance and angle to target the treatment areas effectively.

7. **Comfort**: You'll be positioned comfortably during the session, either sitting or lying down. Red light therapy is painless, and you should only feel a gentle warmth on your skin.

8. **Session Frequency**: The frequency of professional sessions varies based on your skin concerns and goals. Some individuals may benefit from weekly sessions, while others may require less frequent treatments.

9. **Post-Session Care**: After the session, you can typically resume your daily activities immediately. The professional may recommend applying a hydrating moisturizer to lock in the benefits.

What Conditions Can Professional Red Light Therapy Address:

Professional red light therapy can be used to address a wide range of skin concerns, including:

- **Anti-aging**: Red light therapy stimulates collagen production, reducing the appearance of fine lines and wrinkles.

- **Acne**: It can help manage acne by reducing inflammation and promoting skin healing.

- **Rosacea**: Red light therapy may reduce redness and improve the overall appearance of rosacea-prone skin.

- **Psoriasis**: It can slow down the excessive cell turnover associated with psoriasis, providing relief.

- **Eczema**: Red light therapy may help manage eczema symptoms, including itching and inflammation.

- **Wound Healing**: Professionals use red light therapy to promote wound healing and scar reduction.

Cost and Duration:

The cost of professional red light therapy sessions varies depending on factors like location and the expertise of the provider. It's essential to discuss pricing during your consultation. The duration of your treatment plan will depend on your specific skin concerns and goals.

Maintenance and Follow-Up:

To maintain the benefits of professional red light therapy, you may require ongoing sessions. The professional will provide guidance on your follow-up schedule and any at-home care you should incorporate into your routine.

Conclusion:

Professional red light therapy treatments offer a specialized and tailored approach to addressing various skin concerns. Whether you're seeking anti-aging benefits, acne management, or relief from skin conditions, consulting with a skincare professional can provide you with expert guidance and access to high-quality red light therapy devices. Be sure to research and choose a qualified and experienced provider to ensure safe and effective treatments.

Common Myths and Misconceptions: Addressing misconceptions about red light therapy and clarifying its true potential.

Red light therapy is a promising skincare and wellness treatment, but it has also been the subject of myths and misconceptions. Let's address some of the most common misconceptions and provide clarity on the true potential of red light therapy:

Myth 1: Red Light Therapy Is Harmful Like Tanning Beds:

- **Reality**: This is a common misconception. Unlike tanning beds, which emit harmful UV rays, red light therapy uses non-UV red and near-infrared light. It's non-invasive and safe for the skin when used as directed.

Myth 2: Red Light Therapy Is a Fad with No Scientific Basis:

- **Reality**: Red light therapy is grounded in scientific research. Numerous studies have shown its effectiveness in various applications, from skincare to pain management. It's not a passing trend but a well-established practice.

Myth 3: Red Light Therapy Is Only for Skin Beauty:

- **Reality**: While red light therapy is renowned for its skincare benefits, it has broader applications. It's used for wound healing, pain relief, muscle recovery, and even in clinical settings for specific medical conditions.

Myth 4: Red Light Therapy Provides Instant Results:

- **Reality**: While some people may notice improvements after a few sessions, red light therapy is not an instant fix. It often requires consistent use over several weeks or months to achieve significant and lasting results.

Myth 5: All Red Light Therapy Devices Are the Same:

- **Reality**: Red light therapy devices vary in terms of wavelength, intensity, and quality. Medical-grade devices used in professional settings differ from consumer-grade products. It's essential to choose a device that suits your specific needs.

Myth 6: Red Light Therapy Can Replace Skincare Products:

- **Reality**: Red light therapy can complement skincare products but doesn't replace them. Skincare products provide topical nourishment, while red light therapy works at a cellular level to enhance skin health.

Myth 7: It Doesn't Matter How You Use Red Light Therapy:

- **Reality**: The effectiveness of red light therapy depends on proper usage. Factors like session duration, distance from the device, and the specific area targeted all play a role. Following usage guidelines is crucial.

Myth 8: Red Light Therapy Is Only for Certain Skin Types:

  - **Reality**: Red light therapy is generally safe for all skin types and tones. It doesn't carry the risk of hyperpigmentation or other adverse effects associated with some skincare treatments.

Myth 9: Red Light Therapy Has No Side Effects:

  - **Reality**: Red light therapy is considered safe, but like any treatment, it may have side effects for some individuals. These can include mild skin irritation or temporary redness. Consultation with a healthcare professional is advisable for those with specific concerns.

Myth 10: You Can't Use Red Light Therapy with Other Treatments:

- **Reality**: In many cases, red light therapy can be used alongside other skincare treatments or therapies. However, it's essential to consult with a healthcare professional to ensure compatibility and safety.

Conclusion:

Red light therapy is a versatile and evidence-based treatment with various benefits for skincare and overall wellness. By dispelling these common myths and misconceptions, individuals can make informed decisions about incorporating red light therapy into their routines and understand its true potential for improving skin health and well-being.

Potential Side Effects and Precautions: Understanding any potential side effects and when to exercise caution.

Red light therapy is generally safe and well-tolerated, but like any treatment, it's essential to be aware of potential side effects and take precautions to ensure a positive experience. Here's a comprehensive guide to understanding potential side effects and when to exercise caution with red light therapy:

Common Side Effects:

1. **Mild Skin Irritation**: Some individuals may experience temporary skin redness or irritation, similar to mild sunburn. This typically resolves within a few hours to a day.

2. **Dryness or Flaking**: In rare cases, red light therapy may lead to dryness or flaking of the skin. This can be managed with a moisturizer.

Precautions and Considerations:

1. **Eye Protection**: Always wear appropriate eye protection, such as goggles or eye shields, when using red light therapy devices that emit bright light. This prevents potential eye strain or discomfort.

2. **Photosensitivity**: If you are taking medications or using skincare products that make your skin more sensitive to light (photosensitive), consult with a healthcare professional before starting red light therapy.

3. **Pregnancy**: While red light therapy is generally considered safe during pregnancy, pregnant individuals should consult their healthcare provider before starting any new treatment.

4. **Cancer and Tumors**: If you have a history of skin cancer or are currently undergoing cancer treatment, consult with an oncologist or dermatologist before using red light therapy.

5. **Medical Conditions**: If you have specific medical conditions or concerns, such as epilepsy or lupus,

consult with your healthcare provider to ensure red light therapy is safe for you.

6. **Skin Sensitivity**: Individuals with highly sensitive skin or a history of skin allergies should perform a patch test on a small area of skin to check for adverse reactions before using red light therapy on a larger scale.

7. **Device Quality**: Ensure that the red light therapy device you use is of high quality, meets safety standards, and has been approved for home use if applicable.

8. **Consistency**: To minimize the risk of side effects, follow the recommended guidelines for session duration, frequency, and distance from the device. Overuse or misuse may increase the likelihood of adverse effects.

9. **Skin Care Products**: Avoid applying photosensitizing skincare products (those that make your skin more sensitive to light) before or immediately after a red light therapy session.

Consultation with Healthcare Professionals:

If you have specific concerns or medical conditions, it's advisable to consult with healthcare professionals before starting red light therapy. They can provide personalized guidance and ensure that the treatment aligns with your overall health and wellness plan.

Conclusion:

Red light therapy is a safe and effective treatment option for many individuals seeking improvements in skin health, pain relief, and overall well-being. By understanding potential side effects and taking necessary precautions, individuals can enjoy the benefits of red light therapy with confidence and peace of mind.

Long-Term Skin Health**: Strategies for maintaining youthful and radiant skin as part of a lifelong approach to skincare

Achieving youthful and radiant skin is not just about quick fixes; it's a lifelong journey that involves consistent care and healthy habits. Here are strategies to maintain long-term skin health and sustain that youthful glow:

1. **Sun Protection: Shield your skin from UV rays by using broad-spectrum sunscreen with SPF 30 or higher daily, even on cloudy days. Wear protective clothing and accessories like hats and sunglasses when spending time outdoors.

2. **Hydration: Maintain skin moisture by drinking plenty of water throughout the day. Proper hydration helps keep your skin supple and radiant.

3. **Balanced Diet: Consume a diet rich in fruits, vegetables, lean proteins, and whole grains. Antioxidant-rich foods like berries, spinach, and nuts can help protect your skin from oxidative stress.

4. **Avoid Smoking: Smoking accelerates skin aging by damaging collagen and narrowing blood vessels. Quitting smoking can lead to noticeable improvements in skin health.

5. **Limit Alcohol: Excessive alcohol consumption can dehydrate your skin and contribute to skin issues. Enjoy alcoholic beverages in moderation.

6. **Regular Exercise: Physical activity promotes healthy circulation, which can enhance skin tone and texture. Aim for regular exercise to keep your skin looking its best.

7. **Stress Management: Chronic stress can lead to skin problems. Practice stress-reduction techniques such as meditation, yoga, or deep breathing exercises to maintain skin health.

8. **Adequate Sleep: Quality sleep is essential for skin rejuvenation. Aim for 7-9 hours of restful sleep each night to allow your skin to repair and regenerate.

9. **Skincare Routine: Establish a consistent skincare routine that includes cleansing, moisturizing, and protecting your skin. Choose products tailored to your skin type and concerns.

10. **Exfoliation: Include gentle exfoliation in your routine to remove dead skin cells and promote cell turnover. Overdoing it can lead to irritation, so follow product instructions.

11. **Sun Avoidance: Avoid direct sun exposure during peak hours (10 a.m. to 4 p.m.) when UV radiation is strongest. Seek shade or use protective measures when outdoors.

12. **Professional Care: Consider professional skincare treatments such as facials, chemical peels, or red light therapy to enhance and maintain skin health.

13. **Avoid Harsh Products: Steer clear of harsh skincare products that can strip your skin of natural oils and cause irritation. Opt for gentle, pH-balanced formulations.

14. **Consistency: Stick to your skincare routine and healthy habits consistently. Long-term results require ongoing commitment.

15. **Regular Check-ups: Periodic skin assessments by dermatologists can help detect skin issues early and ensure proper care.

16. **Lifelong Learning: Stay informed about skin care advancements, ingredients, and trends. Continuously adapt your routine based on your skin's changing needs.

17. **Healthy Lifestyle: Embrace a holistic approach to wellness. Address overall health through a balanced diet, regular exercise, and stress management.

18. **Avoid Over-treatment: Be cautious about overusing skincare products or undergoing excessive treatments. Less can often be more when it comes to skincare.

19. **Positive Attitude: Maintain a positive outlook on aging and beauty. Embrace the changes that come with age and focus on feeling confident and healthy.

20. **Enjoy Life: Engage in activities that bring you joy and fulfillment. Happiness can radiate from within and contribute to a vibrant appearance.

By integrating these strategies into your daily life, you can nurture long-term skin health and enjoy radiant, youthful skin as part of a lifelong commitment to self-care and well-being.

DIY Red Light Therapy Recipes**: Ideas for creating natural skincare products at home to complement red light therapy.

Creating your own natural skincare products at home can complement the benefits of red light therapy and contribute to healthier, radiant skin. Here are some DIY recipes to try:

1. **Nourishing Face Mask:

  - **Ingredients**:
    - 1 tablespoon of plain Greek yogurt
    - 1 teaspoon of honey
    - 1 teaspoon of turmeric powder (for its anti-inflammatory properties)

  - **Instructions**: Mix the ingredients to form a paste. Apply the mask to your face, leave it on for 15-20 minutes, then rinse with warm water. This mask can soothe and hydrate your skin.

2. **Hydrating Facial Serum:

  - **Ingredients**:
    - 1 tablespoon of aloe vera gel

- 2-3 drops of vitamin E oil (a powerful antioxidant)
    - 1-2 drops of lavender essential oil (for its calming properties)

    - **Instructions**: Combine the ingredients in a small bottle. Apply a few drops to your face after cleansing and before moisturizing. This serum can lock in moisture and provide extra hydration.

3. **Exfoliating Sugar Scrub:

  - **Ingredients**:
    - 2 tablespoons of brown sugar
    - 1 tablespoon of coconut oil (melted)
    - 1 teaspoon of lemon juice (for brightening)

    - **Instructions**: Mix the ingredients to create a paste. Gently massage the scrub onto damp skin in circular motions, then rinse. Use this scrub once or twice a week to exfoliate and rejuvenate your skin.

4. **Calming Redness Relief Toner:

  - **Ingredients**:
    - 1/4 cup of witch hazel (a natural astringent)

- 1/4 cup of rosewater (soothing and hydrating)
- Aloe vera gel (optional, for additional hydration)

- **Instructions**: Combine the ingredients in a spray bottle. Apply the toner to your face after cleansing to reduce redness and promote skin balance.

5. **Anti-Acne Spot Treatment:

  - **Ingredients**:
    - 1-2 drops of tea tree oil (known for its antibacterial properties)
    - 1-2 drops of lavender oil (for soothing)
    - A carrier oil like jojoba or grapeseed oil

  - **Instructions**: Mix the essential oils with a carrier oil. Apply a small amount to acne-prone areas before bedtime. These oils can help address blemishes and calm irritated skin.

6. **Soothing Eye Cream:

  - **Ingredients**:
    - 1 tablespoon of shea butter (moisturizing)
    - 1 teaspoon of almond oil (nourishing)

- 1 teaspoon of aloe vera gel (soothing)

- **Instructions**: Combine the ingredients and gently apply the cream around your eyes. Shea butter and almond oil can hydrate the delicate eye area.

7. **Natural Lip Balm:

  - **Ingredients**:
    - 1 tablespoon of coconut oil
    - 1 tablespoon of beeswax (for texture)
    - A few drops of peppermint essential oil (for a refreshing scent)

  - **Instructions**: Melt the coconut oil and beeswax together, add the essential oil, and pour the mixture into lip balm containers. Apply to your lips for soft, hydrated lips.
8. Soothing Oatmeal Bath:

  - **Ingredients**:
    - 1 cup of rolled oats
    - A muslin bag or clean cloth

  - **Instructions**: Place the oats in a muslin bag or tie them in a clean cloth to create a pouch. Hang the pouch under the faucet while filling your bathtub with warm water. Enjoy a soothing oatmeal bath to calm irritated skin and relieve itchiness.

9. Overnight Hair Mask:

  - **Ingredients**:
    - 2 tablespoons of coconut oil
    - 1 tablespoon of honey
    - 1 egg yolk (rich in protein)

    - **Instructions**: Mix the ingredients until well combined. Apply the mask to your hair, focusing on the ends. Cover your hair with a shower cap and leave it on overnight. Rinse thoroughly in the morning for nourished and shiny locks.

10. DIY Massage Oil:

  - **Ingredients**:
    - 1/4 cup of sweet almond oil (or a carrier oil of your choice)
    - A few drops of your preferred essential oil (e.g., lavender, eucalyptus, or peppermint)

- **Instructions**: Combine the carrier oil with your chosen essential oil. Use this homemade massage oil to relax your muscles or promote overall well-being.

11. Moisturizing Body Butter:

  - **Ingredients**:
    - 1/2 cup of shea butter
    - 1/4 cup of coconut oil
    - A few drops of your favorite essential oil (for fragrance)

  - **Instructions**: Melt the shea butter and coconut oil together, then add the essential oil. Allow the mixture to cool and solidify. Whip it into a creamy texture and apply as a luxurious body butter for deep hydration.

12. Homemade Bath Salts:

  - **Ingredients**:
    - 1 cup of Epsom salt
    - 1/2 cup of sea salt
    - A few drops of essential oil (e.g., lavender, chamomile, or eucalyptus)

- **Instructions**: Mix the salts and essential oil together. Add a few spoonfuls to your bathwater for a relaxing and muscle-soothing soak.

13. Refreshing Cucumber Toner:

  - **Ingredients**:
    - 1/2 cucumber (peeled and blended)
    - 1 tablespoon of rosewater

  - **Instructions**: Blend the cucumber until it becomes a smooth puree, then mix it with rosewater. Apply the toner to your face to refresh and hydrate your skin.

14. Natural Deodorant:

  - **Ingredients**:
    - 1/4 cup of baking soda
    - 1/4 cup of cornstarch
    - A few drops of essential oil (e.g., tea tree, lavender, or lemon)

  - **Instructions**: Mix the baking soda and cornstarch, then add the essential oil for fragrance. Apply this natural deodorant to keep underarms feeling fresh.

These DIY recipes offer natural alternatives to commercial products and can enhance your self-care routine. Experiment with different ingredients and essential oils to create personalized skincare and wellness products that suit your needs and preferences.

Frequently Asked Questions: Providing answers to common questions readers may have about red light therapy.

1. **What is red light therapy, and how does it work?**
   - Red light therapy, also known as photobiomodulation, involves exposing the skin to low-level red and near-infrared light. These wavelengths penetrate the skin's surface, stimulating cellular energy production and promoting various therapeutic effects, including skin rejuvenation.

2. **Is red light therapy safe for all skin types?**
   - Red light therapy is generally safe for all skin types and tones. Unlike some skincare treatments, it doesn't carry the risk of hyperpigmentation or adverse effects associated with UV exposure.

3. **What are the benefits of red light therapy for the skin?**
   - Red light therapy can improve skin health by reducing wrinkles, promoting collagen production, addressing acne, reducing inflammation, enhancing blood flow, and supporting overall skin rejuvenation.

4. **How often should I use red light therapy?**

   - The frequency of red light therapy sessions can vary depending on your specific goals and the device you're using. Typically, starting with a few sessions per week and gradually increasing frequency is recommended.

5. **Is red light therapy painful or uncomfortable?**

   - No, red light therapy is non-invasive and painless. You may feel a gentle warming sensation on your skin during a session, but it should not cause discomfort.

6. **Can red light therapy be used with other skincare products or treatments?**

   - Yes, red light therapy can be used alongside other skincare products and treatments. It can complement your existing skincare routine and enhance the effectiveness of certain products.

7. **How long does it take to see results from red light therapy?**

   - Results from red light therapy can vary depending on individual factors and the specific skin concerns you're addressing. Some people may notice improvements after a few weeks, while others may require several months of consistent use.

8. **Are there any side effects or precautions with red light therapy?**

   - Red light therapy is generally safe, but some individuals may experience mild skin irritation or temporary redness. It's important to follow usage guidelines and consult with a healthcare professional if you have specific concerns or medical conditions.

9. **Can red light therapy be used on other parts of the body, not just the face?**

   - Yes, red light therapy can be used on various areas of the body, including the neck, chest, hands, and larger muscle groups. Many devices offer full-body treatment options.

10. **Is red light therapy suitable for individuals with specific skin conditions?**

    - Red light therapy has shown promise in addressing various skin conditions such as acne, eczema, and psoriasis. However, it's essential to consult with a dermatologist or healthcare professional to determine its suitability for your specific condition.

11. **Is red light therapy suitable for pregnant individuals?**

- While red light therapy is generally considered safe during pregnancy, pregnant individuals should consult with their healthcare provider before starting any new treatment or wellness regimen.

12. **Are there any age restrictions for red light therapy?**
   - Red light therapy is suitable for individuals of various ages. It can be beneficial for both younger individuals looking to maintain skin health and older individuals seeking to address signs of aging.

13. **Can red light therapy be used in combination with other anti-aging treatments like Botox or fillers?**
   - Yes, red light therapy can complement other anti-aging treatments, such as Botox or dermal fillers. It can help promote overall skin health and support the effects of these treatments.

14. **Is red light therapy a replacement for sunscreen?**
   - No, red light therapy is not a replacement for sunscreen. While it can improve skin health and reduce the appearance of wrinkles, sunscreen is essential for protecting the skin from harmful UV radiation.

15. **Can red light therapy devices be used at home?**

- Yes, many red light therapy devices are designed for home use. They are safe and convenient options for individuals who want to incorporate red light therapy into their daily routines.

16. **What are the differences between red light therapy and other light-based treatments like laser therapy or IPL (intense pulsed light)?**
   - Red light therapy uses lower-energy light wavelengths compared to laser therapy or IPL, which are more focused and intense. Red light therapy is non-ablative and non-thermal, making it a gentle and non-invasive option.

17. **Is red light therapy suitable for all skin concerns, or are there specific conditions it works best for?**
   - Red light therapy is versatile and can address various skin concerns, including wrinkles, acne, and skin rejuvenation. However, its effectiveness may vary based on individual factors and the specific condition being treated.

18. **Can I combine different wavelengths of light in my red light therapy session for added benefits?**
   - Some red light therapy devices offer the option to combine different wavelengths (e.g., red and near-infrared) in a single session to target multiple skin concerns

simultaneously. Consult your device's user manual for guidance on wavelength selection.

19. **How can I maintain and clean my red light therapy device for optimal performance and safety?**

- Proper maintenance and cleaning are essential for the longevity and effectiveness of your red light therapy device. Follow the manufacturer's instructions for maintenance, which may include cleaning the device's surface and replacing bulbs when necessary.

20. **Are there any contraindications or specific medical conditions that may require avoiding red light therapy?**

- While red light therapy is generally safe, individuals with specific medical conditions or those taking photosensitizing medications should consult with a healthcare provider before starting red light therapy. Conditions like epilepsy or lupus may require special consideration.

These FAQs provide a more comprehensive understanding of red light therapy, addressing common questions and considerations for those interested in incorporating this treatment into their skincare and wellness routines. Always prioritize safety and seek professional guidance when needed.

Resources and References**: A list of recommended books, websites, and scientific studies for further exploration.

Explore the following books, websites, and scientific studies to delve deeper into the science and applications of red light therapy:

Books:

1. "The Ultimate Guide to Red Light Therapy: How to Use Red and Near-Infrared Light Therapy for Anti-Aging, Fat Loss, Muscle Gain, Performance Enhancement, and Brain Optimization" by Ari Whitten.

2. "The Healing Power of Light: A Comprehensive Guide to the Healing and Transformative Powers of Light" by Primelight.

3. "Red Light Therapy: Miracle Medicine" by Mark Sloan.

4. "Red Light Therapy: Overcome Aging & Fatigue" by Michael Armstrong.

Websites:

1. [National Center for Biotechnology Information (NCBI)](https://www.ncbi.nlm.nih.gov/): Access a vast collection of scientific studies and research articles on red light therapy and its applications.

2. [The Photobiomodulation Society](https://www.photobiomodulation.org/): A resource for information on photobiomodulation, including research, events, and news.

3. [Joovv Blog](https://joovv.com/blogs/joovv-blog): Offers articles, research summaries, and insights into red light therapy for health and wellness.

4. [RedLightMan](https://redlightman.com/): Provides detailed information about red light therapy devices, scientific research, and practical usage tips.

Scientific Studies:

1. Hamblin, M. R. (2017). [Mechanisms and applications of the anti-inflammatory effects of photobiomodulation](https://www.ncbi.nlm.nih.gov/pmc/

articles/PMC5523874/). A comprehensive review of the anti-inflammatory effects of photobiomodulation, including red light therapy.

2. Avci, P., Gupta, A., Sadasivam, M., Vecchio, D., Pam, Z., Pam, N., & Hamblin, M. R. (2013). [Low-level laser (light) therapy (LLLT) in skin: stimulating, healing, restoring](https://www.ncbi.nlm.nih.gov/pmc/articles/PMC4126803/). An exploration of the various applications of low-level laser therapy (LLLT) in skin conditions.

3. Barolet, D., & Boucher, A. (2010). [Prophylactic low-level light therapy for the treatment of hypertrophic scars and keloids: a case series](https://www.ncbi.nlm.nih.gov/pmc/articles/PMC3047738/). A study on the use of low-level light therapy for scar reduction.

4. Calderhead, R. G., & Vasily, D. B. (2013). [Low-level laser (light) therapy (LLLT) for cosmetic medicine and dermatology](https://www.ncbi.nlm.nih.gov/pmc/articles/PMC3799034/). An overview of the applications of low-level laser therapy in cosmetic medicine and dermatology.

These resources and references offer a wealth of information on red light therapy, its mechanisms, and its potential benefits for various skin and wellness concerns. They can serve as valuable sources for those interested in learning more about this innovative treatment.

www.ingramcontent.com/pod-product-compliance
Lightning Source LLC
Chambersburg PA
CBHW062332290526
45794CB00005B/1998